Feeding Yourself
with Love and Good Sense:

Discover the Joy of Eating

Feeding *Yourself* with Love and Good Sense

kelcy press

ISBN 978-0-9671189-9-4

Developmental editor, Nancy Pekar

Part of the five-part series

Feeding with Love and Good Sense: The First Two Years
Feeding with Love and Good Sense: 18 months through 6 years
Feeding with Love and Good Sense: 6 through 13 years
Feeding with Love and Good Sense: 12 through 18 years
Feeding Yourself *with Love and Good Sense*

Show this booklet to your health care provider!

Encourage purchasing in bulk for office or classroom
Discounts up to 50%

Distributed by
Ellyn Satter Institute
www.EllynSatterInstitute.org
esi@EllynSatterInstitute.org

Feeding *Yourself*

with Love and Good Sense:

Discover the Joy of Eating

Ellyn Satter

Nutritionist and Family Therapist

Table of contents

Discover the joy of eating!

This booklet helps you master a kinder, gentler way of eating. It does for you what my colleagues, trainees, and I have often done in our respective practices for people who struggle with eating: help you become eating competent. Being a competent eater is feeling good about eating and doing a fine job with it—being relaxed and confident about taking good care of yourself with food. Throughout this booklet, I am careful to give you permission to eat as much as you want of food you enjoy. If you find the slightest hint of words and phrases that decode as criticism, shaming, or "don't eat so much; don't eat what you enjoy," I hope that you will tell me. I will change them.

Almost everyone has trouble with eating. Your trouble may be smaller or greater. You may already be pretty competent with eating but want to make your eating more rewarding: Make it more of an event, enhance the joy of eating, feel good about eating all kinds of food, solve an eating problem, or develop practical meal-providing strategies. We will do that.

You may struggle enough with your eating that you don't feel relaxed and confident about it. For you, chapter 2 is the core of the booklet, where I help you learn with your body—not your head—to be eating competent. I coach you in physically going through the motions of positive and tuned-in eating. As you give yourself permission to eat and connect again and again with your experience of eating, your eating will transform. The conflict and chaos that you experience with eating will gradually melt away, to be replaced by joy and confidence.

Your struggle with eating may be even more considerable. Colleagues who work with people who have eating disorders observe that this booklet will help, but not right away. In fact, they point out that reading this booklet may bring up issues for you, and even frighten that part of you that depends on tight control with your eating. Chapters 6 and 7 offer resources to help you determine whether your conflict and anxiety about eating could be an eating disorder and give recommendations for seeking help.

Acknowledgements

Ellyn Satter Institute (ESI) faculty members are proficient with healing eating attitudes and behaviors using the eating competence model. They contributed substantially to the content and expertise of this booklet by drawing on their considerable knowledge and skill in family intervention, dietetics, eating disorders, obesity management, diabetes education, health education, psychotherapy, public health, gastroenterology, allergies, sports nutrition, exercise physiology, medical nutrition therapy, pediatrics, and extreme food selectivity.

Anne Blocker, MS, RDN, CSSD, LD, CDCES
Alexia Beauregard, MS, RDN, CSP, LD
Anne Buffington, MA, RDN, CSSD
Peggy Crum, MA, RDN

Carol Danaher, MPH, RDN
Cristen Harris, PhD, RDN, CSSD, CD, CEP, FAND
Jennifer Harris, RDN, LD, CEDRD

Rebeca Hernández, MS, LD
Keira Oseroff, MSW, LCSW, CEDS
Eve Reed, APD
Kerry Regnier, MPH, RDN, LDN

This booklet is also the product of the many minds and much good thinking of friends and colleagues who work with education, journalism, therapy, nutrition, naturopathic medicine, and editing, as well as my daughter Kjerstin and young-adult granddaughters, Emma, Marin, and Adele. They all read from a personal as well as professional perspective, saying what encouraged them and helping get rid of what made them feel bad.

Harriet Brown
Ann Michalski

Jillian Murphy, NMD
Joni Trautman

All who contributed have a wish for you: that you discover the joy of eating. Our very best wishes. Embrace the process. Do the work. Trust yourself to learn and grow.

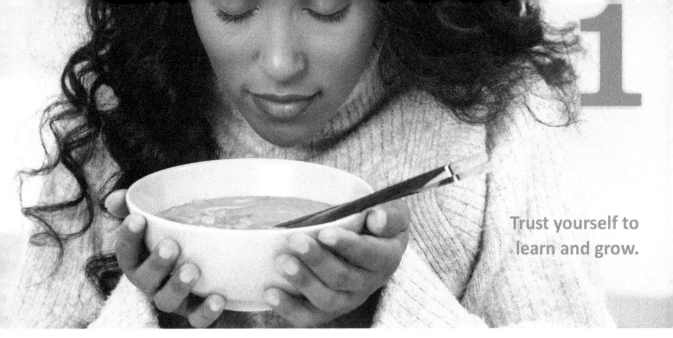

Trust yourself to learn and grow.

How to eat

Would you like to feel good about your eating?

- ❏ Do you often worry about your eating and/or weight?

- ❏ Do you make excuses about your food, about what you eat or how much you eat?

- ❏ Do you feel happy when you eat "good" food and guilty when you eat "bad" foods?

- ❏ Do you try to eat less than you are hungry for?

- ❏ Do you worry that if you eat certain foods you might not stop?

Almost everyone can check at least one of these boxes. In today's world, feeling conflicted and anxious about eating is so common that it may seem the way it is supposed to be. It isn't, and it doesn't have to be that way for you. Checking the boxes does not mean that you have an eating disorder. To know where common upset about eating stops and an eating disorder starts, read chapters 6 and 7.

The goal of this booklet is to help you become a competent eater

- ■ **You feel good about eating**. You enjoy food and feel comfortable eating with others. You look forward to eating rather than being filled with dread or worry.

- ■ **You take an interest in food—even unfamiliar food.** At the same time, you give yourself permission to eat familiar food you enjoy.

- ■ **You eat as much as you want**. You go along with your natural desire to get enough to eat of food you enjoy, rather than fighting against it.

- ■ **You feed yourself regularly and reliably.** Because you enjoy food and feel comfortable with eating, it is rewarding to make feeding yourself a priority.

Competent eating is healthy eating

Why become a competent eater? Let me tell you a story. In the first years of my dietetics clinical practice, I found myself spoiling my patients' eating. When we first met, they were, for the most part, relaxed and comfortable with choosing food, eating, and cooking. Then I put them on a diet: to lose weight, prevent heart disease, manage diabetes, etc. Within a few weeks, they had lost their joy and ease with eating. They had become suspicious of food and no longer enjoyed cooking. Clearly, I was harming, not helping them.

My patients taught me a better way

I stopped *telling* them what and how much to eat. Instead, I started asking them, "How do you go about feeding yourself?" A pattern emerged. People who did well with eating felt good about it, enjoyed all kinds of food, ate as much as they wanted, and fed themselves regularly and reliably. They were competent with eating! I stopped giving diets and, instead, based my nutrition counseling on achieving the pattern of eating

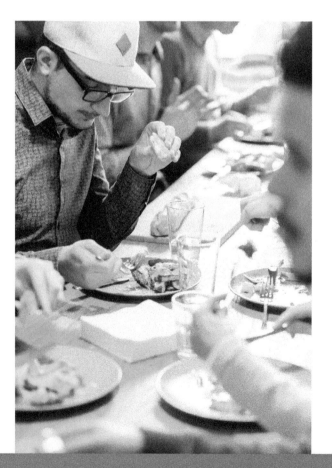

competence my patients had taught me. We had fun together, and they showed the health benefits that they hadn't achieved by struggling with diets.

The Satter Eating Competence Model (ecSatter) and the test: ecSI 2.0™

I wrote a test, ecSI 2.0™, and my patients' scores matched what they told me. High scores indicated that they felt good about eating and fed themselves regularly and reliably. Dr. Barbara Lohse, a creative and rigorous researcher, validated the test for research and determined that the eating pattern my patients and I had developed is nutritionally sound. Since the first publication in 2007, over 20 studies have confirmed and furthered our early results: People who test high on ecSI 2.0™ do significantly better.

- **Medical**. Their blood pressure, blood glucose, and triglycerides are lower and their cholesterol shows a more desirable pattern.

- **Nutritional**. They have both nutritionally adequate and high-quality diets. They eat more fruits and vegetables and whole grains and less fat, salt, and sugar.

- **Body mass index**. Their body weights are stable and often lower, and their weight dissatisfaction and drive for thinness are low.

- **Socially and emotionally**. They are more aware and accepting of how they feel and what they want and, based on their self-awareness, are able to develop satisfying relationships with other people.

Today's food climate is like a diet

Nowadays, people come into clinical offices with their eating already spoiled. Today's food climate is like a combination of all the diets I ever gave and many that I did not. The consequences are just as dire. People have lost their joy and ease with eating and demonize perfectly acceptable food. The solution for you is the same as for my patients. Stop trying to follow lists of dos and don'ts. Instead, focus on allowing yourself to regain your competence with eating. Feed yourself faithfully and give yourself permission to eat.

Discover the joy of eating

This page gives you the big picture of what to do to become competent with your eating, and what to expect as you do it. It may be all you need. Most people need more help, however, and the next chapter gives specific steps to take in becoming eating competent. After you work your way through those chapter 2 steps, this page will make more sense to you.

Feed yourself faithfully

Reassure yourself you will be fed and that you will get to eat food you genuinely enjoy. Having a pattern of meals and snacks supports you in taking care of yourself with food.

- Take time to sit down to eat.
- Develop a meal and snack routine that works for *you.*
- Include foods you *truly* enjoy. Don't let your eating competence be spoiled by lists of good foods and bad foods.

Give yourself permission to eat

Reassure yourself: "It's all right to eat this. I just need to pay attention while I eat."

- Eat what you want. Your body needs variety and your soul needs pleasure.
- Eat as much as you want. Your body knows how much it needs to eat.
- Eat it if it tastes good. Don't eat it if it doesn't taste good.

Feed yourself faithfully

Give yourself permission to eat

This icon reminds you of the keys to joyful eating: Take time to feed yourself. When you eat, give yourself permission by saying, "It's all right to eat this. I just need to pay attention."

Notice as you learn and grow

Becoming competent with your eating is a process, and it takes time. As you feed yourself faithfully and give yourself permission to eat, you will find your eating falling into place.

- You feel good about your eating and are reliable about seeing to it that you get fed.
- You get better and better at eating as much as you are hungry for.
- If you eat fruits, vegetables, whole grains, and other "recommended" foods, you do it because you *enjoy* them, not because you have to.
- You enjoy "forbidden" food, and you are as relaxed about it as every other kind of food.
- Big servings don't make you overeat. You eat it all if you want to, not if you don't.

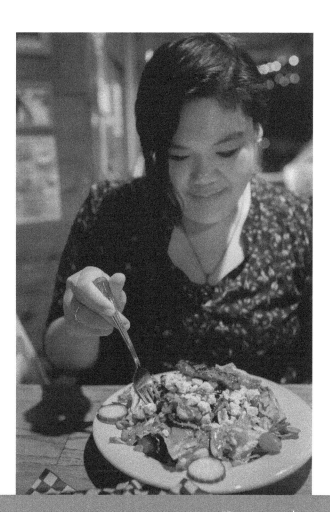

Being eating competent *works*

Ashley didn't know how to feed herself

Ashley's parents had always told her what and how much to eat. When she went away to college, she was so overwhelmed by the choices in the school cafeteria that she didn't eat much all day. Then in the evening she got really hungry and figured this was her treat time, so she ate constantly until bedtime. The dietitian counseled Ashley in being connected with her eating and snacking intentionally rather than munching continually. Ashley got so she could go to the cafeteria without being afraid of binging, and even began to experiment with a few new foods. For the first time and without worry she was able to truly enjoy eating with her friends.

Patty said she was a picky eater

Patty stopped being ashamed that she ate only a few foods. Instead of criticizing herself for eating from a *short* list, she learned to say to herself, "It's all right to eat this, I just have to pay attention." When others criticized her for eating so few foods, Patty found the courage to ask, "Why would you make an issue of what I eat?" Once she got the pressure off herself, Patty likely learned to eat a few more foods. But maybe she didn't. That's not the point.

Sarah was ashamed of liking bread

Sarah felt bad about enjoying bakery-fresh bread. The dietitian told her to give herself permission to eat it, that fresh bread is as good as it gets, bread-wise. Sarah ate it every single meal for at least a month. Then she said, "I don't want any more bread. Bread is okay, but I need something more, like tomatoes and avocados."

Joseph tried not to eat fine-tasting food

After he learned to connect with his eating, Joseph was amazed that he could enjoy fine-tasting food without going on an eating binge. When he was growing up, Joseph's mom was a terrible cook, she made a lot of food, and she insisted Joseph eat it all. Joseph learned to eat a lot whether he wanted it or not and to put himself on automatic pilot to do it. Joseph gained more weight than was right for him when he was a boy and retained that excess weight as an adult. After Joseph learned to eat competently, his weight stabilized, and his blood sugars improved.

Amanda found her stopping place

Amanda was startled to find her stopping point halfway through her second delicious piece of pumpkin pie. She tried a couple more bites, but she truly didn't want any more. Once she realized what she had done, she was ecstatic. "Do you have any idea how good it feels to look at a piece of pie and truly not want it? Knowing there is a stopping point is kinda like sanity."

Elias told the family secret

After he listened to me tell his parents that there had to be a good reason for his sneaking food, 10-year-old Elias told the family secret. Sure, they were finding food wrappers under his bed, but everybody else in the family had a food stash! They all had a good laugh, then addressed the real problem. They were being so righteously "healthy" at mealtime that they were driving themselves to secret eating.

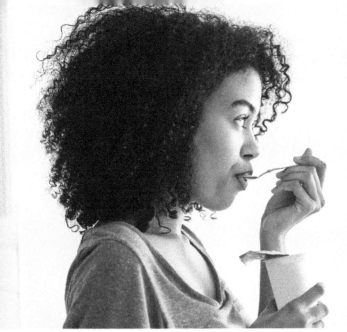

2

Feed
yourself
faithfully

Give yourself
permission
to eat

Learn with your *body*

Discover the joy of eating!

When you go through the motions of feeding yourself faithfully and giving yourself permission to eat, you discover with your very being what healthy and normal eating—competent eating—is all about! You become relaxed, self-trusting, and joyful with eating, and you take good care of yourself with food.

Reassure yourself you will be fed

- Start your day with some idea of when and how you will feed yourself.

- Try for meals but do the best you can.

- Give your comfortable, reliable routine time to evolve. It could take weeks—months!

- Put together meals and snacks with food you *truly* enjoy, not just food you think you *should* enjoy.

> A family meal is when you all sit down together, face each other, and share the same food. Period. It's not about the food you do or don't have to eat.

Give yourself permission to eat all food

- **Be grateful for it**. All food nourishes your body.

- **Recognize its value.** All food gives you protein, energy, vitamins, minerals, and other nutrients.

- **Enjoy it**. Added sugar and fat don't take away nutrients. Canned peaches and fried fish are still—peaches and fish.

- **Relax about it**. Include "forbidden" foods in meals and snacks often enough so you can be relaxed about eating them—and not have to binge to do it.

Start small

- Eat what you eat now.

- Try for meals but don't insist.

- Start by connecting with your eating (next page).

Connect with your eating

Connecting with your eating will transform it. It seems like magic, but there it is. Call it meditation, mindfulness, intuition, attunement, being focused. It's about getting in touch with your inner self—your inner self that knows how to eat.

Feed yourself faithfully

Give yourself permission to eat

Relax and be mindful

Stop, breathe, and say to yourself, "It's all right to eat, I just have to pay attention." The hardest part is remembering to do it! We aren't talking about do-this-all-the-time-for-it-to-work. Do it when you think of it, for as long as you think of it—or can tolerate it. At first, two or three bites will be enough for you to remember and/or tolerate it. As your comfort increases, you will connect for more and more bites until you find your yourself connecting through much of the meal or snack. So . . . here we go. Get your food lined up. Carve out some time. Sit down . . .

Take a breath or two.
In through your nose (slow count of three).

Out through your mouth (slow count of three).

(Did you forget? Pause and take your breaths when you think of it.)

Tune in to your food.
How does it look?

How does it smell?

What is going on inside you?

Pay attention to your mouth.
Take a bite. How does it taste and feel?

What goes on inside you?

Swallow when you feel like it.

Wait to get the next bite ready until after you swallow.
Look at the food as you put it in your mouth.

How does it taste and feel?

What goes on inside you?

Swallow when you feel like it.

Eat as much as you want. Your body knows how much to eat.

Connect with what lies inside you

Feed yourself faithfully

Give yourself permission to eat

As you connect with your eating (previous page), connect with yourself. Ask yourself, "What am I experiencing while I eat?" At first you may just get self-talk that *interferes* with connecting. You may worry about what or how much to eat or whether giving yourself permission will affect your weight. That self-talk gets in the way of your knowing what goes on inside you—your hunger, appetite, and feelings of reward and satisfaction from eating. As time goes on, you will be less and less bothered by that self-talk and more and more, longer and longer, be tuned in to your inner self while you eat.

What is your payoff?

Ask yourself, "What payoff am I getting from tuning in?" You may be more tuned in to yourself and your circumstances of eating. You may get a glimpse of feeling better about your eating: calmer, or more tuned in. You may feel a bit more comfortable about providing yourself with food. Repeatedly asking yourself this question will help you keep track of how your eating is changing. Be careful *not* to say, "If I do this, I won't eat so much." That is building in a punishment and is an example of destructive and undermining self-talk.

Make peace with what lies inside

With awareness comes change. As you connect with your eating, you will encounter feelings and memories—even strong and painful ones. Tune out if it is too much. Tune back in when you are ready. Feeling and remembering, again and again, lets you gain comfort with your feelings and memories. Gaining comfort lets you relax and enjoy eating.

Consider your feelings—and your feelings about your feelings

- Enjoying eating. Feeling excited. Being ashamed of your excitement.
- Feeling upset and turned off. Feeling upset about being turned off.
- Feeling afraid of not getting enough to eat. Feeling upset about being afraid.

Consider how tastes and smells take you back

- Sweet memories of people and places. Missing them.
- Upsetting memories of people and places. Not wanting to remember.
- Negative memories of being shamed about your eating.
- Anxiety that seems to come from nowhere.

Have an intentional snack to practice connecting with your eating

Keep this practice session short: a couple of minutes. Choose a small amount of food you really enjoy: a cookie, some chips, a little piece of bread and jam, or maybe just a couple of bites of something. The idea is to connect all the while you eat without having it feel overwhelming. This is about connecting. It is *not* chew-it-40-times-before-you-swallow or chew-it-until-it-loses-its-texture-and-becomes-liquid (ugh!).

- Breathe.
- Look at your food.
- Give yourself permission to eat.
- Take a bite.
- Pay attention to your mouth.
- Swallow when you feel like it.
- Look at your food.
- Prepare the next bite.
- Stop when the food is gone.

Trust your body to know how much to eat

It could be that you are way ahead of me. You have already discovered that your body knows how much to eat. If not, you will. This page addresses in more detail supporting yourself in knowing how much to eat.

Feed yourself faithfully

Give yourself permission to eat

Say to yourself, "It's all right to eat *as much as I want*. I just have to pay attention."

- Choose food you enjoy.
- Go to eating times hungry but not starving.
- Pay attention while you eat.
- Eat as much as you want.
- Stop when you feel like it.
- Take a few more bites to be sure.
- Stop.
- Remind yourself: "I can do this again—and again."

You will get in touch with your body

Trying to ignore and outwit your body lets you feel only the strongest feelings—being famished or being stuffed. At first you may not feel hungry when you start or full when you stop. Keep your nerve! If you avoid sipping and munching between times, your hunger rhythms will adjust to your eating pattern. Then you will recover more subtle feelings—maybe a twinge of hunger; maybe a bit of fullness, but not really being sure. Your feelings of hunger and fullness will get stronger. Then you will rediscover your stopping place.

Keep your nerve about your weight

If you deprive to force your weight down, you will gain it back. If you overeat to force your weight up, you will lose it back. When you first connect and give yourself permission with eating, your weight may be a bit variable, especially if up to this time you have been undereating or overeating. Courage! Your weight will stabilize. Your body is wise. It "remembers" and adjusts by being more or less hungry and by burning off more or fewer calories. That *remembering* is powerful and even *unstoppable*. You get hungry, you eat, you become satisfied, you stop eating. You eat a lot today, this week, this month, and even this *season*, and less another.

Are you in touch with your hunger?

The irony, in this land of plenty, is that hunger bothers us, not because we can't afford to buy enough food, but because we continually try to undereat. Becoming competent with eating lets you feel differently about hunger. As you gain comfort and confidence with your eating, you will more often check the first box in each section.

How do you feel when you are hungry?

❑ Excited.

❑ Afraid.

How do you feel when you are eager to eat?

❑ Pleased.

❑ Ashamed.

How do you feel when there is lots of food?

❑ Relieved.

❑ Threatened.

How do you feel when you are full?

❑ Comfortable.

❑ Like you have to work it off.

❑ Like you have to get rid of it.

Trust your body to eat what is good for you

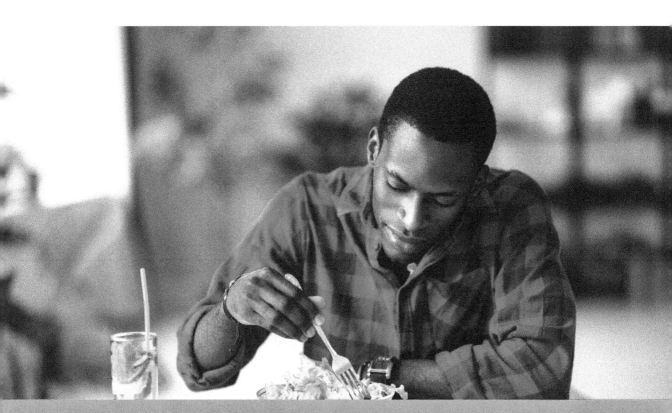

When you first start feeding yourself faithfully and giving yourself permission to eat, you may eat the same food all the time, food you haven't let yourself eat before. Enjoy it! You may—in fact, you must—give yourself permission to eat food you enjoy and keep on giving yourself permission.

Don't let this next bit scare you

This is what will happen for you. It is not what is *supposed* to happen or what you have to *make* happen. It is an important difference. I am teaching you about the natural process of growth and development with food acceptance that you will experience as a competent eater. I am not telling you what you *should* do, which is the opposite of being a competent eater.

You will tire of even your favorite foods

Remember Sarah and her bakery-fresh bread (page 4)? Sarah ate it every meal for a month, then got enough of it and became interested in tomatoes and avocados.

In some ways, that story would be more freeing if Sarah developed an interest in French fries or cupcakes and let herself eat them. Her turning to tomatoes and avocados seems like saying, "How Sarah grew up and learned to eat her vegetables." But there it is. Sarah truly enjoyed tomatoes and avocados. Once she got enough of her fresh bread, she discovered that other foods appealed to her, as well.

How will this play out for you?

You may eat your same favorite foods every meal, every day, for *months*. Years, even. That's just fine. It is exactly what you need to do. You have spent a long time feeling you shouldn't eat those foods. You need a long time to feel good about eating them. Eventually you will find, like Sarah did, that you are losing interest in your same favorite foods and beginning to feel like experimenting with other food.

Ever so gradually, you will increase your variety

You will increase the variety of food you enjoy because you want to and feel like it, not because you should.

What learning to trust yourself with eating looks like

Let's imagine that you are in my office. I coach you in giving yourself deliberate permission to eat: "It's all right to eat. I just have to pay attention." That is shorthand for "Feed yourself faithfully; give yourself permission to eat." I encourage you to have meals, but also warn you not to do too much, too soon. Get started by giving yourself permission to eat whenever you eat, whether you are reading or walking or leaning on the kitchen counter. As you go along, a meal-and-snack rhythm will emerge.

We set up a series of appointments. Each time you come back to see me, I ask, "What did you find out about your eating?" At first, you are caught in your head, wondering about what food to eat or not-eat, what to have for meals. You might plead for a diet. These are the ways your thoughts and fears get in the way of your tuning in on your relationship with food. Instead of addressing these thoughts and fears, I ask you, "What did you notice about what goes on inside of you?" At first, you draw a blank. But after a few weeks, you talk less about your food rules and anxiety and more about your hunger, appetite, response to the food, and the feelings, sensations, and memories that come up for you when you pay attention to your eating.

I say, "Let's keep on, and see what more you find out." Each week, you feel more and more calm, comfortable, peaceful, and satisfied. You even comfortably eat "forbidden" food! You rarely binge, and then it doesn't seem like a binge and more like just eating a lot! Then, one day, you come in excited about finding your stopping place. You were enjoying a meal or snack and discovered you genuinely didn't want to eat any more. You did a few experimental bites to be sure. And you stopped eating, knowing there was another meal or snack coming when you could do it all over again.

Then we celebrate. And I hide my tears. It is so moving for me to share in your epiphany.

Do you need in-person expert help with learning to eat?

You can go through the steps in this chapter by yourself, or you can do it with someone else you trust. Sharing your hang-ups and discoveries about eating with another person can help you be more relaxed and accepting of how you think and feel. That person can be a calming presence when you are upset and remind you to get out of your head and into your body when you get trapped by the food rules. But you do need in-person expert help if you are exceptionally bothered, rigid, or immobilized with your eating. A qualified professional can evaluate whether you have an eating disorder and design treatment that is specific for you.

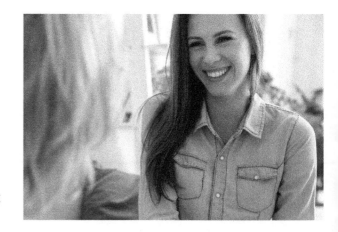

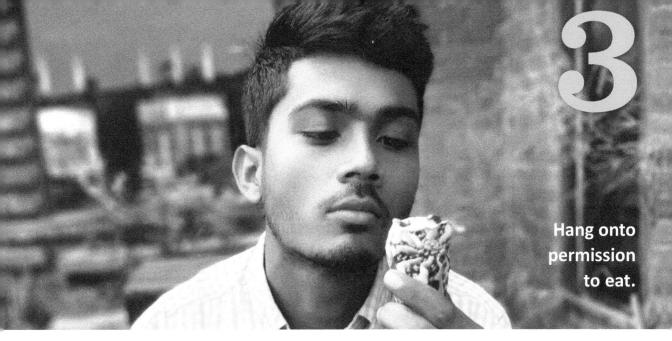

3

Hang onto permission to eat.

Resist interference

In chapter 2, you learned to trust yourself with your eating. This chapter is about protecting yourself so you can hang on to your competence with eating. Negative messages about eating, food and weight are all around. Learn to identify and ignore these messages. They can undermine your being a competent eater. Let's start with the negative messages you impose on yourself.

Perfectionistic thinking

While connecting with your eating will form the basis for your sense of comfort and order with eating, there will be times when you want to eat fast or absent-mindedly. Let yourself be flexible. There is more than one way to eat. You can decide: Which manner of eating is best *right now*? What manner of eating is best over the long term?

Eating binges

Binging is different from letting yourself eat fast or absent-mindedly because binging feels so self-destructive. Consider what happens. Does it feel like there are two of you, one who wants to eat, the other who says, "don't eat?" Do you try to ignore them both, then cut loose, and eat? That's not all bad. At least, the "I want to eat" part gets to eat! But the "don't eat" part scolds and punishes. Instead, why not say to yourself, "I feel like eating a lot, and that is okay." "I feel like vegging out with a bowl of popcorn in front of the TV, and that's okay."

Saying "don't eat that."

Were you thinking "I shouldn't eat that," "that's too fattening." Or were you indulging in weight talk? You know, "I'm too fat." "Maybe that diet will work for me." Getting into diet thinking is traumatic. The trauma is all the negative feelings that go along with food restriction: being constantly hungry; being preoccupied with what to eat or not eat; being demoralized when your weight stays the same. Going on automatic pilot with your eating is your escape. You don't need that. Remember, it is okay to eat what and as much as you want.

Don't get tangled up in rules

Rules take away your joy of eating, cast doubt (and guilt) on your cherished family foodways, and create roadblocks to your becoming and remaining competent with your eating. We are up to *here* with food rules: Eat this. Don't eat that. Eat to neutralize or compensate or detoxify.

Being a competent eater lets you eat enjoyably and well

Feed yourself faithfully; give yourself permission to eat. Remember, people who are positive, joyful, and reliable with eating—who are competent eaters—do better medically, nutritionally, emotionally, and socially.

Official dietary guidelines

The dietary guidelines are much the same in every country: Emphasize vegetables and fruits, eat whole grains instead of refined, eat low-fat meat and not much of it, use low fat dairy, limit sugar, salt and fat. Exercise a lot. We translate the guidelines into rules and health professionals, the media, even *fiction* for goodness sake, harp on them. You don't need rules in order to eat the food you need. Trust yourself to eat what and as much as you need. Let yourself learn and grow with food acceptance.

Clean eating

Clean eating goes farther than the dietary guidelines, saying to have unprocessed whole foods, whole grains, lean meats, and no artificial ingredients, preservatives, "chemically-charged foods," sugars, saturated fats, and trans fats. Clean eaters even feel bad about eating fruit because it "is nothing but sugar." There is at yet no research addressing health outcomes of clean eating.

Consider the rules that tangle you up

You may eat vegetarian or even vegan, or follow a Paleo, gluten-free, or low-carbohydrate diet. You may be committed to organic, locavore, or low-carbon (footprint) eating. Your food rules may be a hodgepodge of any or all of the above as well as dos and don'ts from every magazine article you have ever read and every diet you have ever been on.

Consider how food dos and don'ts make you feel

Guilty? Self-critical? Immobilized? Most people have a vague set of rules, at least enough to feel "I know I should, but . . . " Having a big gap between what you think you *should* eat (or do or feel) and what you *do* eat (or do or feel) makes you feel bad. Feeling bad about your food is not a basis for competent eating.

Consider the bottom line

Your food rules may make you feel secure. Following a diet may show you how to feed yourself. It may help you act on your values. But here's the deal: Are you enjoying eating? Is eating a chore or a bore? Do you have to take vacations or plan cheat days to get away from the rules? The positive benefits of being a competent eater likely grow out of *consistency*. To be consistent and reliable about taking care of yourself with food, enjoy your eating. Feed yourself faithfully and give yourself permission to eat.

Beware of counterfeit permission

- **Controlling messages harm.** They take away permission to eat and make you feel negative and wary about your eating.

- **Permission-giving messages help**. They encourage you to trust yourself with eating.

You can't always tell the difference

Some harming messages are so cleverly disguised they seem to be helping messages. They encourage you to eat less and less-appealing food. They are counterfeits. Such messages may trick your head, but they don't trick your body. In the long run, controlling tactics make your eating unpleasant and send you out of control.

Messages that harm by taking away permission	Messages that help by giving permission
Before you eat, be careful of what goes on your plate.	Eat food you enjoy.
Enjoy your food, but eat less.	"It's all right to eat. I just need to pay attention."
Fill up by drinking water before a meal.	Reassure yourself that you will get enough to eat.
Eat off a smaller plate.	Eat until you feel satisfied.
Pay attention to portion size.	Have as many helpings as you want.
Arrange to run out of fattening food.	Make enough to have leftovers.
Eat sweets in small amounts.	Savor sweets and eat until you get enough.
A cookie is a sometime food.	"C" is for cookie.
Make half your plate fruits and vegetables.	Eat foods you enjoy.
Eat in moderation.	Eat a lot if you want to.
Don't keep "tempting" foods around.	Stock your pantry with food you enjoy.
Cook with recipes that use little sugar, salt, and fat.	Use sugar, salt, and fat to make your food taste good.
Chew every bite carefully.	Pay attention to how good the food tastes.
Cut cheese and chocolate into small pieces and only eat a few.	Savor cheese and chocolate, and you will get enough.
Avoid buffets.	Trust your body to guide you at buffets.
Don't have seconds. If you do, wait 20 minutes first.	Eat as much as you are hungry for.
Serve food portions no larger than your fist.	Eat as much as you are hungry for.

Use—don't abuse—emotional eating

To make positive choices in life, you have to know how you feel. *Using* emotional eating is when you know how you feel and deliberately use food and eating to address those feelings. It is completely and unquestionably natural to use food for emotional reasons. Cooking, eating with friends, and eating by yourself can raise your spirits when you are low, soothe you when you are tense, and distract you when you are upset. *Abusing* emotional eating is when your feelings go straight to eating. You have the impulse to eat but tell yourself it is wrong. You put yourself on automatic pilot and eat-without-eating. That would be eating without paying attention or connecting in any way with your food. You end up feeling anesthetized, or guilty, or out of control.

Do a good job with eating for emotional reasons

As a child you may have learned to connect feelings with eating if your grownups regularly gave you food handouts to entertain you, calm you down, or head off a temper tantrum. While that makes a strong connection between your feelings and eating, it doesn't mean you are doomed. It just means you have to make an effort to sort it all out.

- Know what you feel.

- Ask, "What am I trying to do for myself with this food?"

- Give yourself permission: Reassure yourself that you can eat if you want.

- Consider other ways to take care of yourself: Talk with a friend, take a walk.

- Awareness means choice. Do something else if you want. Eat if you want. Just eat in a way that truly feels encouraging, soothing, or diverting.

How to use, not abuse, emotional eating

- Gain comfort with your feelings and memories. Experience them again and again until they aren't so scary and overwhelming. Get help if you need it.

- Feed yourself regularly and reliably. Being too hungry increases the impulse to eat for emotional reasons.

- Don't try to restrict your food intake. People who eat less than they need tend to abuse emotional eating.

- Understand the sequence. Restricting yourself takes a lot of energy. Stress undermines your energy, you throw away restriction, and you eat. Since you can't deliberately let yourself eat as much as you want, you throw away all controls and eat a lot.

Using emotional eating doesn't make you gain weight

Your body knows how much you need to eat. Even if you deliberately eat a lot for emotional reasons, you will be less hungry the next meal, the next day, or even the next week. This just happens. It doesn't work if you try to force it. But if you abuse emotional eating and then try to make up for it by eating less, it will set up an overeat/restrict cycle that keeps on going and is likely to make your weight unstable.

You don't have to be ashamed of your eating

- ☐ Are you passionate about food?
- ☐ Do you love eating and love the taste of good food?
- ☐ Do you really enjoy "fattening" food?
- ☐ Do you feel you eat more than other people do?

Feel and do *your* way

If you checked any or all of the boxes—*good*! If you didn't, also *good*. People have all sorts of natural and normal ways to feel and do with eating. The problem is that our attitudes about eating are so distorted that being enthusiastic about food and eating, and eating a lot, are considered sure signs that we will gain weight. They aren't. Parents do the best they can, but they pick up on social attitudes and pass them along to their children. Attitudes about eating that you get from your parents are particularly powerful. Can you see yourself in any of these stories?

Sophia *loves* to eat

Five-year-old Sophia loves to eat. She *moans* when she eats. Her father is alarmed. He is afraid that Sophia's enthusiasm for eating is just not *right* and will make her fat.

Even though Sophia's appetite is wonderfully sensitive and compelling, it can be satisfied. She will get enough and stop eating—even when her food tastes so good that it makes her moan. However, she is learning to be ashamed of her appetite. That can make it hard for her to eat much as she needs and could confirm her father's worst fears. She could get too fat.

Arthur is small and doesn't eat much

Seven-year-old Arthur's parents see him as being tiny and worry that he doesn't eat much. They encourage him to eat and even cheer and give him rewards when he eats.

Even if Arthur doesn't eat much, it is enough for *him*. Some children are naturally small. Some children naturally don't eat much, even if they aren't small. However, Arthur is learning to go by what his parents say rather than what his body tells him to determine what and how much to eat. That will make eating unpleasant for him and make him eat even less.

Gracie wants the "wrong" food

Ten-year-old Gracie's parents worry that she is overweight and try to slim her down with food restriction. Gracie tries to cooperate when her parents tell her to eat her chicken and vegetables before she can have rice and bread. But vegetables make her gag. Broccoli is the worst.

Rice and bread are no more likely to make Gracie fat than chicken and vegetables. Restricting her rice and bread makes Gracie want them all the more and feel ashamed for wanting food her parents don't want her to want.

Consider Satter's division of responsibility in feeding

Parents are relieved when they learn Satter's division of responsibility in feeding: It is their job to manage the *what*, *when*, and *where* of *feeding*. It is their child's job to do the *how much* and *whether* of *eating*. It is especially challenging for parents to trust the big- or small-eating child and/or the fast- or slow-growing child to manage whether and how much they eat. But parents do it, and children become competent with eating and grow in the way that is right for them.

Consider your body's wisdom with weight

Your body will regulate if you let it—or in spite of what you do to it. Your body's powerful regulatory systems allow you to maintain a more-or-less stable pattern of body weight. Look back over your last year. In spite of all the different ways you have lived, eaten, drunk, and exercised, your weight is highly likely to have stayed pretty stable or returned to a fairly stable level, despite ups and downs.

Consider a vacation from restricting

Trying to get yourself to eat less and less-appealing food in order to keep your weight down keeps you from being competent with eating. If you have been preoccupied with weight your whole life, giving it up is a tall order. Don't think *forever*; think *right now*.

- Stop trying to lose weight until you get a solid feel for the freedom and sheer pleasure of being a competent eater.

- See what happens with your weight. It will probably be about the same as when you started, maybe a little higher at first. If you have been dieting, it will probably go back to its pre-dieting level.

- Then decide: Are you willing to give up the joy of eating in order to try to lose weight?

The "freshman 15" is really five and it is natural

What did you weigh when you graduated from high school? Have you been trying to maintain that weight ever since? Trying to prevent your natural weight gain will make you fatter, not thinner. Chances are, it was difficult from the first. You were fighting your body's powerful inborn growth drive. Even after high school and into their twenties, boys get taller, and both boys and girls naturally gain an average of five pounds. Teens who diet gain considerably more weight than those who do not. As a woman, your prized body weight might have been in your early teens, when you first got breasts and hips, and the rest of you was still lean. It was nice while it lasted, but your body still needed to grow. Between ages 14 and 18 years, the average girl grows an inch and puts on 15 pounds. And they are good pounds, made up of muscle and bone and, yes, fat. You are, after all, female. The average boy grows 4 inches and gains 20 pounds between ages 14 and 18 years.

Consider what holds true about your dieting

When did you start dieting? How much weight did you lose? Did you gain it back? When did you diet again? What happened after that? Make a graph. What would you predict for your weight if you go on still another diet? It is up to you whether you will step off the dieting merry-go-round or try still again for weight loss.

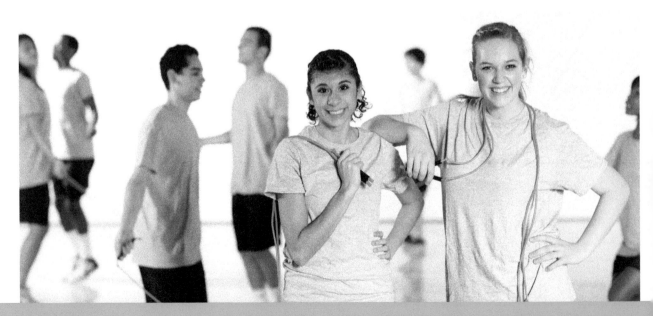

Consider your body's wisdom with activity

Almost everyone can check at least one of these boxes. In today's world, activity is often virtue and obligation, something you do to compensate for eating. While it is healthy to be active, and it does burn off calories, you can't trick your body. It remembers the activity-induced deficit and you are hungrier later on. It's all about attitude. Why not change your attitude about activity? Why not do the same for your activity as you have done for your eating, and consider movement as a source of pleasure and nurturing?

How do you use activity?

☐ To control your weight.

☐ To burn off calories.

☐ To feel in control of your life.

☐ To get the right numbers.

☐ To be healthy.

☐ To improve your mood.

It's all right to move—any way you want and when you are ready

Move because you enjoy it and to enrich your life. You can find activity that feels good and is so satisfying that you keep doing it, the same as with your eating.

- Do you need to move? Consider walking, running, biking, or swimming. Do you need to move in a group? Consider Zumba or aerobics.

- Do you need to feel productive? Consider commuting by walking or biking, gardening, or housecleaning.

- Do you need fun and silliness? Consider playing catch or tag.

- Do you need stillness and connection with yourself? Consider yoga and tai chi.

- Do you need to feel strong? Consider weightlifting or Pilates.

- Do you need to feel coordinated and graceful? Consider dance or barre.

Activity can support eating competence

Moving your body for pleasure—even a bit—helps you become and remain a competent eater.

- It makes your sensations of hunger and fullness stronger and easier to detect.

- It lets you know and trust your body.

- It gives you a sense of vitality and comfort in your body.

- It lets you know and appreciate your body's wisdom, endurance, flexibility, capability, and strength.

Memories and feelings may get in the way

Your feelings and memories may make it hard for you to know that your body wants to move. Hang in there! Feeling and remembering, again and again, takes away the sting.

- Being sweaty and out of breath and finding that yucky or alarming.

- Being bored or dreading activity so much it ruins your day.

- Thinking "no pain, no gain," being miserable the next day, and giving it up.

- Remembering being teased or ridiculed. Feeling bad about being picked last for games.

- Feeling guilty about giving up on fitness programs or weight loss endeavors.

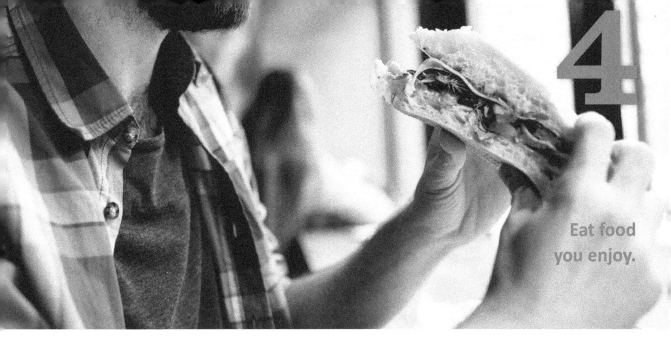

Eat food
you enjoy.

Get the good-food-bad-food monkey off your back

Being competent with eating means that you can eat all food and all kinds of food. But the good-food-bad-food monkey can send you out of control when you want to eat candy or chips or—you name it! It can make your eating unpleasant by obligating you to eat food you *don't* enjoy in the name of health.

Include "forbidden" food

Yes, I really mean it! You may even eat as much as you want of "forbidden" food. You might refer to it as unsafe, feared, or unhealthy food. Whatever you call it, it is high-fat, high-sugar, relatively low-nutrient food such as sweets, chips, and sodas. If you check even one of these boxes, you will benefit from a "forbidden" food attitude adjustment.

❑ Is "forbidden" food your *bad* food—food you crave?

❑ Do you eat "forbidden" food only when you are being *bad*?

❑ Do you eat "too much" when you are being *bad*?

❑ Do you feel guilty about eating your *bad* foods?

❑ Do you try even harder to avoid your *bad* foods, and crave them even more?

Give yourself permission to connect with your "forbidden" food

Go *with* your craving, rather than struggling *against* it. You will calm down and the food you fear will turn into—well—food. Rather than being a big temptation or a no-no, sometimes you want it, sometimes you don't. At first you may eat a lot, but soon the newness will wear off and you will eat less sometimes, more another, the same as you do other food.

- Eat sweets and savory snacks regularly at meal- and snack-time. Connect with your food.

- Reassure yourself: You may eat as much as you want of "forbidden" food.

- Have dessert. Eat dessert first if you want it then.

- Have chips or fries along with your sandwich.

- Have chips and soda, or cookies and milk, for your sit-down snack.

You can feel good about eating food you enjoy

For you to connect and feel positive about your eating, the juice has to be worth the squeeze. Your food has to be rewarding in order for you to go to the trouble of planning, preparing, and eating it. The good-food-bad-food monkey can make you miss out on food you enjoy and make you force down food that you *don't* enjoy in the name of health. It's not good for your body to keep yourself in turmoil about eating.

Appetite is compelling, but it can be satisfied

Enjoy your food. What an alarming notion! Surely if we get the idea that it is okay to enjoy food, we will gobble every unhealthy morsel we come across. And worst of all, we will gain lots of weight! Not so. Getting pleasure from your food is essential in order for you to relax about eating and know you have had enough to eat. Eating a whole package of rice cakes won't satisfy if you really want chocolate chip cookies—or vice versa. You know from experience that you will still eat the cookies!

Connect with eating: You will get enough

At some point you begin to lose interest. Food stops tasting as good. Your interest might drop suddenly or gradually. Eat a few more bites. Keep eating if you are still interested, not if you aren't. As one competent eater put it, "I am ready to stop when my mouth is finished as well as my stomach." Another said it is "a feeling of nuffness."

Include at least one tasty food

Not everyone is a gourmet cook and not every meal can be a masterpiece. But every meal needs at least one food that you truly enjoy. If the main dish is humdrum, include a dessert or bread that is delicious. If the vegetables are tired, go to extra trouble with the main dish. Use condiments to make food taste good. Use butter. It makes good food taste even better. Use salt and your other favorite spices, seasonings, and condiments. Use sugar to brighten the fruit or take the edge off the tomatoes.

Make sure there is enough

Being afraid there isn't enough to go around will positively ruin your meal. If the main dish seems skimpy or the vegetables on the short side, have plenty of bread and rice to fill up on. Yes, I really mean bread and rice. It is a myth that high-carbohydrate foods are fattening. They are bulky and chewy and help you know you have had enough to eat.

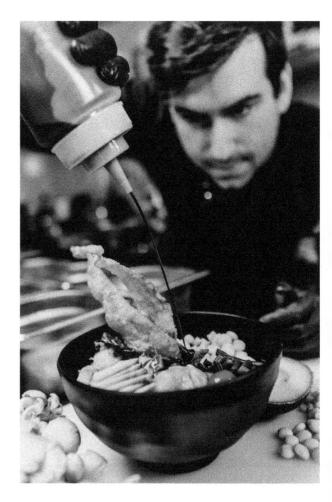

There's nothing to be gained from forcing yourself to eat fruits and vegetables

Consider eating a food you enjoy. Do you look forward to it? Do you start to salivate? This is the *cephalic* phase of digestion. Your mind anticipates eating the food and your body responds. Now imagine knowing you have to eat something you don't enjoy or that even tastes unpleasant. Do you look forward to it? Do you start to salivate? Probably not. Forcing yourself to eat something you dislike stalls digestion because it triggers your body's stress response. Your mouth gets dry, it is hard to swallow, your stomach may feel upset, you might even get diarrhea or become constipated.

Give fruits and vegetables a break

They taste good (to many people), they look pretty, they add variety, and they contribute to health and a nutritionally adequate diet. The problem is the idea that eating them is *desperately* important. How can we possibly learn to enjoy fruits and vegetables when we feel pressured to eat them? Stop forcing. Take a break. In the meantime, remember that you might eat *some* vegetables: think potatoes (French fries). Don't forget tomatoes (pizza and spaghetti sauce). You could even throw in a few onions, peppers, or mushrooms. But don't spoil the dish for yourself! To be a life-long vegetable-eater, you need to *enjoy* them.

What if you *want* to eat fruit and vegetables?

Do you *really* want to, or do you just *want* to want to? Take plenty of time saying *no* to fruits and vegetables (or any other food you don't enjoy) before you let yourself say *yes*. How will you know you are ready?

- Are you getting tired of eating the same foods all the time?

- Are you becoming interested in other foods?

- Would it be easier and more convenient if you enjoyed a few vegetables or fruits?

Here's how to experiment with eating fruits and vegetables

- **Sneak up on them**. Look a little (in the store), buy a little, cook a little, throw away a little.

- **Taste**. Don't make yourself swallow. Take it out again. Repeat . . . repeat . . . repeat . . .

- **Add flavor to vegetables**. Think pumpkin pie. Baked potato with sour cream. Broccoli with cheese sauce. Green bean casserole. Caesar salad with real dressing and Parmesan cheese. Raw vegetables with ranch dip.

- **Make fruit into dessert**. Consider pies and cobblers with ice cream or whipped cream. Canned fruit in heavy syrup. Fresh fruit sprinkled with sugar or coconut.

- **Add salt, fat, and sugar**. Add salt and butter to cooked vegetables. Add bacon. Put a teaspoon of sugar in peas and tomatoes. Use *real* salad dressing.

- **Consider juices**. Juices have all the nutrients from the fruit or vegetable and even some of the fiber.

No meal is perfect: Eat together, anyway

Researchers asked parents what gets in the way of family meals. Here is what they said:

- It's hard to plan ahead and have the time to make a healthy meal.

- We don't sit down and eat together if it's fast food, like we would if it was home cooked.

- Lack of time is number one. That's when the fast food comes in and everyone eats on their own.

What happens when families "eat on their own"

Here's what it might look like. Burgers and potato chips on the counter, each family member shows up to get the food when it occurs to him or her and eats on their own. Chicken nuggets and French fries in the back seat. Pizza for the kids in front of the TV, parents eat when they think of it or when they prepare something for themselves that they enjoy more. How do *you* eat when you don't make it important? That would be eating-without-eating—grabbing what is available; eating it while you study or commute or shave or put on your makeup; being surprised when the food is gone.

"Healthy" is food you enjoy

Many people feel the same as the survey parents, that food has to be "healthy" to make it a meal. But what is "healthy"? *Healthy* is what we have been saying all along: food you enjoy. *Healthy* is food you eat without getting hung up on good-food-bad-food.

Eat what you eat now and know that it is *healthy*

Round up the food and the family, sit down together, share it, and enjoy your time together.

- Hamburgers and chips on the table or on the counter, with plenty to go around.

- Chicken nuggets and French fries sitting at a table in the fast-food restaurant.

- Pizza in the living room for the whole family, watching TV on Friday night. This might interfere with tuning in on eating, but let's be realistic. Movie night is *special*!

Be considerate without catering

Broiled chicken breasts and broccoli with no butter may be your favorite meal. Others may not agree. Here is how to interest others in showing up to eat with you:

- Make your meal filling and still easy to prepare by adding bread, rice, or other starchy food.

- Give your meal staying power and more flavor by having high-fat side dishes: butter, regular salad dressing, hollandaise or cheese sauce.

- Eat what tastes good to *you* from the meal. Even if you planned it and prepared it, you can't predict what will taste good at any one meal on any one day.

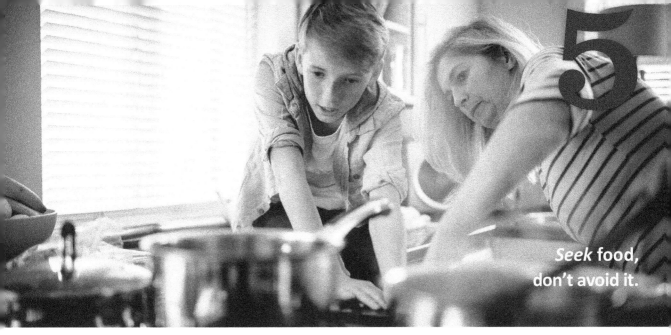

Seek food,
don't avoid it.

Develop strategies for getting fed

Reassure yourself that you will be fed

Once you feel comfortable with *how* to eat, *what* to eat will fall into place. At that point, use this chapter in the way that is right for you. You may develop an appetite, so to speak, for these ideas about managing. You may enjoy planning, shopping, and cooking and use it for fun and relaxation. On the other hand, you may want to do as little as possible to get the job done. However you feel about it is okay.

Be deliberate about feeding yourself

- **Get your food lined up**. Go to some trouble to get food *you* want to eat. Don't wait until you are hungry to think about it, or you will just grab something that you might not enjoy.

- **Pay attention to cravings**. You don't have to give in to every eating impulse but *do* pay attention to cravings that keep coming back.

- **Set aside your food.** Be sure your food will be there, waiting for you. Label it and put it in a special place. Hide it, if you have to.

- **Remember: It's nobody else's business what you eat**. The kids have a saying, "Don't yuck on my yum." You like what you like. It is just plain bad manners to criticize another person's food.

- **Observe yourself developing pride and comfort in your eating**. You will give off "don't bug me" vibes. Or *stop* giving off "criticize me" vibes. Either way, others will know that your eating is off limits.

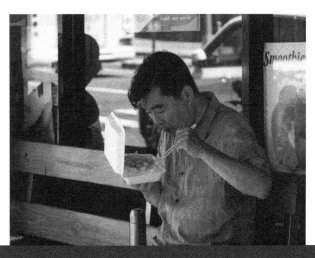

Know why you don't want to have meals

To do a good job with feeding a child, you must have meals. Children are a captive audience, and they need to know they are going to be fed. But for yourself, you can think about it. Are there reasons that you don't want to have meals? It is important to honor your feelings.

- **You don't enjoy mealtime food**. People often eat meals for duty and eat between times for pleasure. The solution? Eat food you enjoy at mealtime. Food you enjoy is likely to be good for you.

- **Meals are a drag**. Were your childhood meals unpleasant? Did people scold and fight? Were you forced to eat more or different food from what you wanted? You can make different choices for yourself. You certainly don't have to force your child to eat.

- **You don't have time**. Meals do take time. Would you take time for meals if the food were good and you could enjoy having a pleasant time?

- **You eat on demand**. You continually ask yourself, "Am I hungry? What am I hungry for?" Did you learn to eat this way to address out-of-control eating? Good for you! Now that you can give yourself permission to eat, why not add structure? Knowing when you will be fed can increase your peace and comfort. It can also let you forget about eating between times.

- **You don't want to be bothered**. If you don't bother with eating, eating will bother you! Whether you know it or not, it scares you to wait until hunger drives you to eat. It makes you grab whatever is available. Knowing you have a meal or a snack coming reassures you that you will be fed and gives you time to think about what you want to eat.

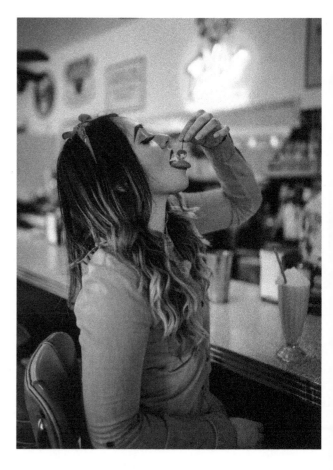

Start by eating what you eat now

Pizza makes a fine meal, so do chicken nuggets or a hamburger and French fries. Just have them at meal- or snack-time, sit, and enjoy them. Put the peanut butter, dill pickles, bananas, jelly, and bread or crackers on the table, and make the sandwich to suit you. Throw in some milk and you have a meal. If the shock of drinking milk is too great, drink what you are drinking now.

Use snacks to support mealtime

Mealtime works best and is most rewarding when you are hungry and ready to eat, but not so hungry you can't wait. Have a sit-down snack to tide you over. Try not to spoil your meal by munching or sipping along between times—except for water.

Mastering meals

- Consider it a meal whether it is defrosted in the microwave, delivered to your door, ordered at a fast-food restaurant, pulled out of a bag, or cooked from scratch.

- Make your meal an occasion. Push back the clutter to give space for your food. Make it pretty if it pleases you. Give yourself permission. Pay attention.

- If you share meals with others, round them up to eat together. Talk and enjoy each other. Don't scold or fight.

- Let your body tell you what and how much to eat from what you have provided for the meal. Avoid pressuring yourself or anyone else to eat. Don't restrict.

Add on, don't take away

Once you get the meal habit, as a competent eater you will learn and grow nutritionally. Tuning in on your eating, you will notice getting tired of eating the same food all the time and start looking around for variety. You will find yourself taking an interest in food, being more comfortable with unfamiliar food, and gradually—ever so gradually—getting so you enjoy a few new foods. The idea is to allow variety without spoiling a good thing.

- Add on to what you usually eat, don't take food away.

- Go slowly and make only one or two changes at a time. You may want to have broccoli and ranch dressing with the pizza. Or have canned peaches with the chicken nuggets and French fries.

- Be considerate without catering. Have only one main dish, then include one or two foods that everyone generally eats. Match unfamiliar food with familiar, not-so-enjoyed food with popular food.

- Plan to eat good-for-you food because you enjoy it, not because you have to.

If you are feeding a family

Starting with familiar foods means family members are likely to be comfortable with the meal. However, don't expect them to eat. You have done your job by providing the meal. Just say (and *mean* it), "You don't have to eat. Just keep us company for a few minutes while we eat."

You will begin to plan a bit

Do you find yourself thinking in the morning when you will carve out time during the day to eat? Do you check the pantry and freezer to figure out what to have for dinner? You are planning. Use planning to reassure yourself. You will be fed and you will get to eat food you enjoy. Knowing what you will eat for a few days and shopping from a list saves time and gives a sense of food security.

Make planning your servant, not your master

You use planning to make it easier to feed yourself. You abuse planning when you make your meals complicated and pile on so much work you can't sustain the effort or when you say, "Oh, I shouldn't eat that. It isn't good for me."

- Include shortcuts. Use convenient foods and ingredients (page 28).

- Use the food groups to help outline meals: meat or other protein; a couple of starchy foods, fruit or vegetable or both; butter, salad dressing, or gravy; and milk.

- Regularly include foods you consider to be "forbidden" food.

- Plan your escape. At times, life gets way too busy and planning will feel too hard. Go back to eating what is easy and familiar. Remember, even the most ho-hum meal is better than no meal at all.

Be cautious about virtue

You do not have to eat food that sucks the happiness out of your mouth. Too often, people who get organized with meals get caught up in the food rules.

- Virtue is eating vegetables and whole grains because you *should*, not because you enjoy them.

- Virtue is condemning perfectly acceptable food for somehow being "unhealthy."

- Virtue is being "good" and then sneaking off for rewards or relief.

It is your business what you eat

Ordinary food from the ordinary grocery store is nutritious, wholesome food. It is a luxury with respect to time and money to choose only organic food, locally grown food, fresh fruits and vegetables, unrefined grains, or foods with no artificial ingredients, hormones, preservatives, sugars, or saturated fat, or food that is salted, smoked, or cured. It is your business what you choose. Prioritize pleasure and consistency. Instead of investing so much in food avoiding, why not put your creativity and energy into seeking new foods or preparing food in new ways?

Do you want more cooking advice?

"How to cook" in *Secrets of Feeding a Healthy Family* helps you find doable ways to build your

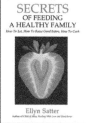

meal habit. Simple and delicious recipes, method summaries, recipe notes, and ideas for cooking with children make this a great book for learning to cook without getting caught in the food rules.

Use strategies that support food regulation

Plan meals and snacks that include carbohydrate (sugar and starch), protein, and fat. Consuming these major nutrients together lets them work best nutritionally and makes meals more satisfying and sustaining. All of us, but some of us in particular, benefit from such well-selected meals and snacks. The active person benefits from the long-lasting energy. The person with heart disease benefits from avoiding getting too hungry, then flooding the system with fatty acids. The person with diabetes benefits from a slow and prolonged release of nutrients that balances with the available insulin and avoids spikes in blood sugar that can overwhelm available insulin.

How nutrients behave in your body

- **Sugar** gets to you quickly and relieves your hunger in a hurry. But it is digested and absorbed quickly so a sugar-only meal, such as soda, fruit, or juice, will soon leave you hungry. Sugar highs and lows and negative behavior have to do with being *hungry*, not from being hyped up by sugar.

- **Starch** has to be digested before it can get to your body, so starch takes longer to satisfy and sticks around longer. A starch-only meal (with a small amount of protein) would be dry bread or bagels, oatmeal, rice, potatoes, or quinoa.

- **Protein** takes even longer to digest and therefore stays in your body even longer than starch. A protein-only meal would be egg white and *very* lean fish. Skim milk has protein and sugar. A sugar, starch, and protein meal would be orange juice, dry toast, and egg white. Since most protein foods also have fat, they last longer because of both the protein and the fat.

- **Fat** stays in your stomach longer and takes longer to digest. Fat can be butter, cream, or real salad dressing, or the fat can be in milk, cheese, meat, poultry, and fish. Read package labels to see if meat and milk substitutes contain fat.

- **Putting all the groups together** gives you a meal or snack that satisfies you quickly and keeps you satisfied for a few hours until the next meal or snack. Think pizza, tacos, tapas, hamburgers, sushi, stir-fry, curry, wraps. The table below may give you more ideas.

Satisfaction from consuming sugar, starch, protein, and fat

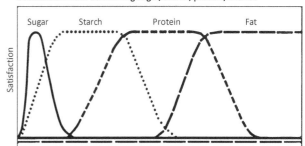

Protein and fat	Carbohydrate	Fat
- 2% or whole milk	- Bread, buns, bagels, taco shells, tortillas, pancakes	- Dips (regular, not low-fat)
- Meat, fish, poultry	- Oatmeal, quinoa, millett	- Butter or cream
- Eggs	- Breakfast cereal	- Cream cheese
- Cheese	- Crackers	- Chips
- Deli meat	- Pastry, cinnamon buns, cookies, cakes, muffins*	- Salad dressing
- Peanut butter	- Popcorn	- Oils, added or used in frying
- Bean dip	- Baked or fried* snacks	
- Hummus	- Raw, canned, or dried fruit	
- Nuts	- Raw vegetables (a bit)	
- Whole or 2% yogurt	- Fruit or vegetable juice	
- Cottage cheese with 4% fat	- Flavored coffee drinks, soda	

*Also have fat

Consider convenient foods and ingredients

Convenient foods and ingredients may or may not be worth the extra expense, depending on whether your time or your money is in shorter supply. Using convenience foods certainly is less expensive than eating out. But remember, the proof of the meal is in the eating. Does it taste good? Is it filling? Is it sustaining? If so, it is a good meal.

Meat, poultry, fish, dry beans, eggs, and nuts

Chicken thighs, boned chicken breasts or stir-fry; canned chicken. Frozen fish fillets, canned tuna or salmon. Boneless pork chops, cutlets, or stir-fry; pork tenderloin; small ham roasts and slices. Beef stew meat (needs to be cooked slowly); breakfast steaks (thin, quick-cooking steaks); prepared beef patties. Regular and low-fat luncheon meats, sausages, and hot dogs. Canned baked beans, cans or jars of precooked navy beans, garbanzos, black beans, and refried beans. Eggs. Peanut butter.

Alternatives: Read labels on vegan meat substitutes. Three ounces (90 grams) should have about 20 grams protein and at least 5 grams fat.

Milk, yogurt, and cheese

Pre-shredded cheese, cheese slices, cheese spread in jars. Milk to drink. Instant and prepared puddings and custards. Plain and flavored yogurt. Canned cream soups to reconstitute with milk.

Alternatives: Read labels for non-dairy soy, almond, rice, and oat beverages to see if they give the same nutrients as dairy milk. A cup of dairy milk has 8 grams protein, 225 mg calcium, 100 IU Vitamin D, and 0, 5, or 8 grams fat depending on whether it is skim, 2%, or whole milk.

Vegetables

Frozen potatoes, instant mashed potatoes, dry packaged scalloped potatoes. Canned or frozen vegetables. Prewashed salad fixings, shredded coleslaw mix, shredded carrots, peeled baby carrots. Vegetable juices, such as tomato and vegetable juice cocktail.

Fruits

Fresh, canned, or frozen fruits and fruit juices. Pre-washed and portioned fruits from the produce section. Fruit nectars (apricot nectar is a good source of vitamin A). Dried fruits such as raisins, prunes, apricots, apples, peaches, mangos, figs.

Breads, cereal, rice, and pasta

Use enriched or whole grain. Sliced bread, buns. Noodles, macaroni, spaghetti. Ramen noodles. Rolls, frozen bread dough, corn bread mix, muffin mix, biscuit mix, pita bread, tortillas. Canned biscuits or rolls. Instant white or brown rice. Quinoa. English muffins, bagels. Pancake mix. Focaccia. Dried packaged or frozen rice, pasta, or bean meals.

Sauces and seasonings

Ingredients you can keep on hand let you put together quick and tasty meals from ready-to-go foods. Think of prepared sauces such as spaghetti or pizza sauce, cream soups, and seasonings to sprinkle on (lemon pepper), to mix in (taco mix), or to serve on the side (salsa, tartar, or cocktail sauce).

Find a prepackaged meal that is *a meal*

You may discover prepackaged meals that work for you. You will learn by experience when a meal has enough calories to fill you up and stay with you for 3 or 4 hours. Unless your energy needs are unusually low, a diet meal won't do it. Consult the nutrition label for food composition information. A meal needs protein, fat, and carbohydrate. Here's what to look for, per serving:

- 15-20 or more grams protein.

- 20 or more grams fat.

- 30 or more grams carbohydrates.

Be an eating-competent vegetarian

There are many good reasons for eating a vegetarian diet, but weight loss isn't one of them. Striving for weight loss by any means compromises your competence with eating. Meat, and to a much lesser degree, poultry and fish are much maligned, but in reality, they have much to offer nutritionally: high-quality protein, of course, as well as B6, B12, niacin, zinc, and iron. Including dairy products and eggs helps fill in nutritional gaps, but you still have to address getting enough calories and iron. If you follow a vegan diet, work with a dietitian to be sure you don't develop a B12 or other nutritional deficiency.

Putting together a nutritionally adequate meatless meal

- **Protein.** Have dried beans, peas, lentils, nuts, seeds, nut butters, tofu, or soy-based meat substitutes to get iron as well a protein. Eggs, milk, and cheese give protein.

- **Grains and starchy foods.** Choose enriched or whole-grain breads, rice, and noodles to give iron. Look for breakfast cereal that offers 40-45% of the daily iron requirement.

- **Fruit or vegetable or both**. Canned, frozen, fresh, 100% juice, or dried all give vitamins and minerals, including iron. Increase your absorption of iron from other food by having orange juice, tomatoes, or another good vitamin C source with meals.

- **Milk.** Use whole or 2% milk to provide fat. Read labels to find almond, rice, soy, oat, or other dairy substitutes that have as much protein, calcium, and vitamin D as milk. Since plant-based beverages are likely to be low in fat, be sure to include fatty foods with meals.

  - **Fat.** Use fat at meals to compensate for low-calorie vegetarian food, and let your appetite guide you in how much to eat. Consider using butter, margarine, salad dressing, or oil in cooking. Add vegetable dip, sauces, gravy, and avocado. Use fat in cooking.

Consider becoming a flexitarian

You can have the best of both worlds. If you are a carnivore, have an occasional—or regular—vegetarian meal as a way of exploring other foods and adding variety and nutritional value to your diet. If you are a vegetarian, be flexible in the other direction: Add small amounts of meat, fish, or poultry to a legume-based dish. In either event, you will stretch food dollars and add nutritional value.

Combine limiting amino acids

There are good nutritional reasons behind traditional vegetarian dishes: The science of complementary proteins. You need a combination of nine essential amino acids to build and repair body tissues. Animal-based protein foods have them all. Plant-based proteins are high in some amino acids, lacking in others. Over the ages, cooks have learned to put together the amino acid jigsaw by using food with high levels of one amino acid to make up for another food with low levels. You don't have to eat complementary proteins at the same meal; eating them in the same day will do. These ideas will get you started.

Legumes + Grains	Legumes + Seeds
- Bean or split pea soup and crackers	- Hummus (chickpea and sesame seed dip)
- Peanut butter on wheat bread	- Sunflower seeds sprinkled on navy bean soup
- Black beans and rice	- Falafel patties with tahini (sesame butter)
- Corn tortillas and refried beans	- Snack mix of roasted soybeans and seeds
- Tofu and bulgur (wheat)	

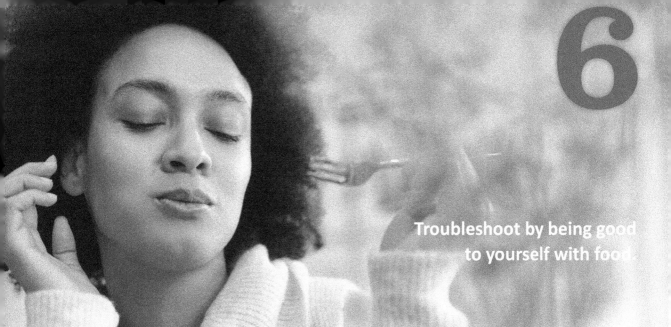

6

Troubleshoot by being good
to yourself with food

Solve eating problems

I am ashamed of how much I eat

You can only know how much you *need* to eat by how much you *do* eat.

Why do you think you eat too much— or too little?

Is it because you eat more or less than other people do? Is it because you are fatter or thinner than you want to be? Is it because others comment on your eating? We address weight dissatisfaction later in this chapter. For now, know that if your weight is stable, you eat the right amount for you. You only eat too much if you gain weight without stopping, or eat too little if you lose without stopping. Of course, that doesn't happen—even for people who are very fat or very thin. Eventually weight gain or weight loss levels off.

Did you grow up feeling you ate too much or too little?

When children are unusual in any way, parents try to nudge them toward the usual. It is what parents do! Here is what we wish your parents had known about your eating:

- One child eats more—or less—than another. A 6-year-old could eat from 500 to 5000 calories a day, an adolescent up to 9500 calories!

- Children eat more one day or at one meal than they do at another.

- Children stop eating when they are full, even if they eat a little or a lot—even if it is ice cream!

- From birth, some children are just naturally big—or small. Many adolescents plump up before they get taller. As long as growth is consistent, that is okay.

- You can't know by looking how much a person eats. Many fat people don't eat much, and many thin people eat a great deal.

I am a really picky eater

We all have food preferences. We eat what we eat. If all goes well, we also have ways of sneaking up on new food and learning to eat it. However, you are *stuck* with your food preferences if you:

- Get upset when you are offered unfamiliar food.

- Only, ever, eat from a short list of foods.

- Worry whether you will be able to eat when others control the menu.

- Feel ashamed of what you eat.

Consider your history

Did this start when you were a child? Did your parents try to get you to eat certain foods, and you simply couldn't do it? You may have angrily refused, but under it all you likely felt ashamed. The same as other children, you wanted to please your parents, and you simply *couldn't do it*. When you became an adult, your parents' attitudes and expectations became your own. Now you apply pressure and feel ashamed all by yourself. Why not give yourself a break?

Give your blessings to the food you eat right now

Yes, I really mean it: *the food you eat right now.* Forget about what you *should eat*. Choosing food based on shoulds and oughts puts pressure on your eating and makes you feel ashamed and anxious. Neutralize your shame and anxiety by giving yourself permission to eat the foods you enjoy. Once you calm down, you may learn to eat new foods. You may not. The important change is letting yourself enjoy eating. Read *Eating competence with food acceptance* on the next page.

- Reread page 5 about developing a mealtime routine. Everything applies to you and the food you eat *right now*.

- Follow the directions on page 7 to connect with your eating. Keep in mind that is the *food you eat right now.*

- Reassure yourself: You don't have to eat anything you don't want to eat.

- As it says on page 7, connect with what lies inside you. You may need help from a skilled professional to stay calm, connected, and self-aware while you eat.

Learn good manners with eating

You don't have to eat with others if you don't want to. You are ready to eat with others when you are comfortable with your own eating and when you can defend yourself against unwanted attention. You will find the courage to ask, "Why would you make an issue of my eating?" But you can't afford bad manners. They attract attention, and you don't need that!

What is okay

- Picking and choosing from what is on the menu. Ignoring the rest.

- Declining to be served.

- Eating only one or two food items.

- Leaving unwanted food on your plate. Resign from the "clean plate club."

- Taking modest helpings, and more of one food when you haven't finished another.

What is not okay

- Drawing attention to your food refusal.

- Asking for food that is not on the menu.

- Eating someone else's share.

- Commenting on your own or someone else's eating.

I wish I enjoyed more foods

Consider your food history. You may have been exposed to few foods, pressured to eat, or even expected to eat foods that upset you or made you sick. You don't have to do the same to yourself as an adult. Instead, trust yourself to eat what you want and not eat what you don't want. Your desire to learn and grow will push you along to learn to enjoy a greater variety of food.

> ## Raise a child who feels good about eating
>
> Follow Satter's division of responsibility in feeding (sDOR). sDOR shows you how to do a good job with feeding by taking leadership with the *what, when,* and *where* of *feeding* and trusting your child to manage the *how much* and *whether* of *eating.*

Eating competence with food acceptance

I hope your work in chapter 2 has let you feel better about eating. Reassure yourself that you don't have to eat anything you don't want to. Be flexible in your thinking. What does food acceptance look like when you are a competent eater?

- You are comfortable with providing yourself with food you enjoy, including food that is high in fat, salt, and sugar.
- You are calm in the presence of food, including unfamiliar and disliked foods.
- You are able to pick and choose from available foods, politely and matter-of-factly accepting or turning down what is offered.

It's up to you whether you experiment

Be absolutely clear about this: Do you *really* want to learn to enjoy unfamiliar food, or do you just *want to* want to? You likely have been selective about food for a long time, so it may take a long time to get ready to experiment. Be patient with yourself. Trust your feelings, don't get pushy, move along at your own speed, and only experiment when you are *really* ready. Here is how to sneak up on new food:

- Look, but don't buy.
- Watch others eat. Help prepare it.
- Buy a little (a very little). Prepare but don't eat.
- Taste but don't swallow.
- Swallow but don't eat more.
- Keep doing it. It will take dozens of unpressured tries.

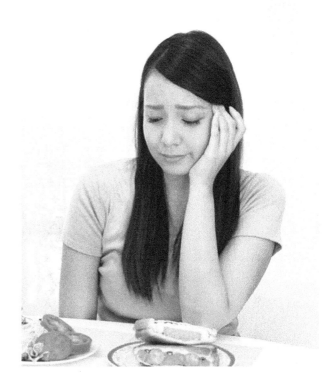

I can't lose/gain weight

You deserve to know the sorry facts about weight. Our national conviction that thinner is better—and that it is achievable—is simply wrong. Health policy says that "normal" weight is average weight or below. That classifies most of us as too fat, whether or not we really are. Popular opinion does the same. What is seen as ideal weight is actually below-average weight, making most of us feel too fat. What about being too thin? Since thin is the body ideal, does your feeling "too thin" mean that you have exceptionally slim muscles, or unusually slender breasts and hips?

Why not be good to your body?

What will it take for you to give up pursuing weight loss? Do you have to be beaten up again and again by losing weight and then gaining it all back? Or are you ready to give it up? While 99.9% of us don't look like fashion models or sports stars, we do perfectly well with our lives. Our bodies take us where we need to go, and we find success and joy in life. Instead of worrying about your weight, why not let yourself enjoy the respect for your body that grows out of being a competent eater? Are you willing to sacrifice that amazing sense of achievement and those marvelous feelings in order to try to lose weight? Why not replace your dream of being thinner with the reality of being all you can be, just as you are?

Trying for weight loss can make you fatter

The biological pressure to regain lost weight is simply enormous. You might be able to keep your weight down for a while, but it will bounce back when you can no longer tolerate undereating and over-exercising. Weight loss cycling can get you into the yo-yo effect and make you fatter than is natural for you, stair-stepping up after each attempt to lose weight. While we know less about thin people who repeatedly try to gain weight, your own life experience will tell you. It is incredibly difficult to change the weight your body prefers.

Health and weight

Optimism, self-trust, and a sense of adventure are healthier for you in guiding your eating than negativity, self-denial, and avoidance. When you are competent with eating, your weight will be and remain right for you, even if it is higher than "normal." You might even weigh a bit less. People who are competent with eating do weigh less, as demonstrated by research studies with women and men of varied income levels, people with diabetes, and college and high school students. Not only that, but studies show that, irrespective of BMI, those who are eating competent have healthier blood lipids, blood pressure, and blood glucose. They even have better oral health! Also keep in mind that the health consequences of high body weight have been much exaggerated. It is simply not true that having even considerably above average weight will make you sick or kill you early. Yo-yo dieting is the real culprit, as it contributes more to illness and early death than stable but high weight. Yo-yo dieters have more heart disease, diabetes and insulin resistance, gall bladder disease, bone fractures, and depression.

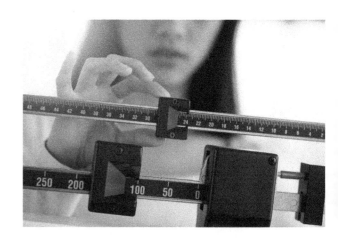

I have trouble eating a healthy diet

What does "eating a healthy diet" mean to you? Avoiding sugar and fat? Avoiding gluten? Avoiding additives, pesticides, genetically modified crops, milk produced using growth hormone, or milk in general? Do you think in terms of altruism or the health of the planet and avoid factory-farmed eggs, chicken or pork, and feedlot raised beef? Do you hope that eating a "healthy" diet will give you a good memory and steady nerves, clear skin, a smoothly functioning liver and colon, and regular and pain-free menstruation? Are you concerned about avoiding chronic disease, such as cancer or heart disease? It is a lot, isn't it? And it all has to do with demonizing food, the antithesis of being a competent eater.

Find a balance

I won't argue with altruism, and it is understandable to try modifying your diet in hopes it will help address ill-defined and hard-to-manage medical problems. Just know that if the dietary modification doesn't help, and especially if your eating becomes more negative than positive, it is time to seek help from an eating-competence savvy professional. You can both address your concerns *and* continue to be a competent eater.

Being eating competent supports wellness

While food avoidance to maintain health and prevent degenerative disease doesn't work, being a competent eater supports good health. Competent eaters do better medically and nutritionally, have stable body weights, and feel good about their bodies.

Eating competently encourages eating a nutritionally adequate diet made up of a wide variety of food that has been tested over the millennia to be safe and incorporated into tried and true foodways. Variety supports health and dilutes any naturally or artificially occurring food toxicants. There is more: Competent eaters are more active, sleep better, and have higher overall social and emotional functioning. With eating, as in life, competent eaters are tuned in and responsive to information coming from within and use that information to guide them in taking care of themselves.

How does your eating make your spirit, mind, and body feel?

- Are you tuned in, relaxed, and comfortable about choosing, preparing, and eating your food? If so, you are supporting your emotional health as well as the smooth functioning of your digestive tract. Being afraid to eat makes your entire digestive system tense up, and it doesn't function as well.

- How do you feel when you finish eating? Steady? Comfortable and relaxed? Fueled? Getting enough to eat is calming and lets you forget about eating for a while.

- How do you feel when you have enjoyed your food? Cheered up? Supported? A satisfying meal feeds the spirit as well as the body.

- Do you enjoy eating with other people? Are you confident you can eat in public? Getting caught up in food avoidance interferes with your emotional and social functioning.

I have trouble managing my eating for diabetes I and II/prediabetes

If you are a competent eater, you are doing your very best to manage your prediabetes or diabetes. In fact, everything about taking good care of yourself with food in every chapter of this booklet applies to you. You can eat as much as you want of food you enjoy. You just need to pay particular attention to maintaining structure.

It's all about balance

Having prediabetes or diabetes means your body has access to only so much insulin at one time. This is true whether you are managing with diet alone, taking medication to help your body make more insulin, or injecting insulin. Structure helps you balance your food intake with your available insulin and your activity to keep your blood sugar within a stable range that lets you feel good. Skimping at one meal and overdoing it at another gives you lows then highs in blood sugar. Losing weight then gaining it back does the same.

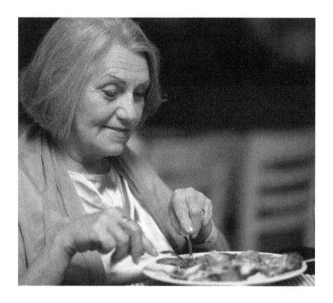

Instead of food avoidance or restriction, think *strategy*

Check your blood sugar and pay attention to how you feel. Too-low blood sugar can make you feel shaky. Too-high blood sugar can make you feel listless and even nauseated. If your blood sugar is consistently too low or too high, talk with your health care professional about adjusting your medication.

Level off your routine

- Have good-tasting, filling, and sustaining meals and snacks. For more detail, see the table and explanation, *How nutrients behave in your body* (page 27).

- Slow down blood sugar release from desserts, soda, and other sweets by consuming them at mealtime, with other food. Make choices about your beverage intake based on your blood sugar readings.

- Review *Consider your body's wisdom with activity* (page 17). Regular movement is a powerful ally in helping your body use insulin effectively.

Why you can't follow your diabetes eating plan

How realistic is it for you to lose weight? Can you always be on a diet, eat a certain amount of food every day, follow a particular pattern for meals and snacks, and exercise a certain amount? Maybe so, but most people go on and off their regimen, feel bad, and have poor average blood sugars and A1Cs. And get pep talks: "If you stay on your diet you won't have to take insulin." Maybe, maybe not. Becoming competent with eating might or might not help you avoid going on insulin. Try to see injecting insulin as a positive step, not as a failure. The nature of diabetes is that your body has less and less ability to produce insulin as time goes on. Injecting insulin may let you feel better and make it easier to manage your diabetes.

I have food allergies

As difficult as it is, it is good to take care of yourself by avoiding foods that you truly can't have. It is not good to be enslaved by a list of allergy maybes. To tell the difference, get a diagnosis from an allergist, and challenge with the offending food under medical supervision. If your symptoms are hard to pin down and possibly psychosomatic, consider a blind challenge, where the offending ingredient is disguised. Seek guidance from a food allergy specialist dietitian on what foods you need to avoid and what foods you can include.

Begin by building a strong foundation of being a competent eater

It is all too easy to focus so much on what not to eat that you become super-sensitive about food, anxious about eating, and overly restrictive with food choices. Seek help from a professional who will support and preserve your eating competence and has experience working with people who have food allergies. Together you can rebuild your eating, following the principles we have emphasized throughout this booklet.

- Start from the foundation of regular meals and snacks.

- Incorporate enjoyable food you find acceptable. Avoid your allergenic foods.

- Connect with your experience of eating.

The competent eater with allergies

You can address your food allergies and still feel good about and be comfortable with eating:

- **Attitude.** You look forward to eating rather than being filled with dread or worry.

- **Food acceptance.** You take an interest in food and have a gradually expanding list of enjoyable and acceptable food.

- **Food regulation.** You go along with your natural desire to eat as much as you want of acceptable food that you enjoy.

- **Managing your food context.** Because you enjoy your food and feel comfortable with eating, it is rewarding for you to make feeding yourself a priority.

Food insensitivities or intolerances

Food sensitivities are food reactions related to your immune system, and even harder to pin down. Intolerances relate to digestive issues, for instance, inability to digest lactose (milk sugar), or celiac disease caused by true gluten intolerance. As we said earlier, get help finding what holds true for you. It is good to take care of yourself by avoiding foods that you truly can't have. It is not good to be enslaved by a list of food maybes.

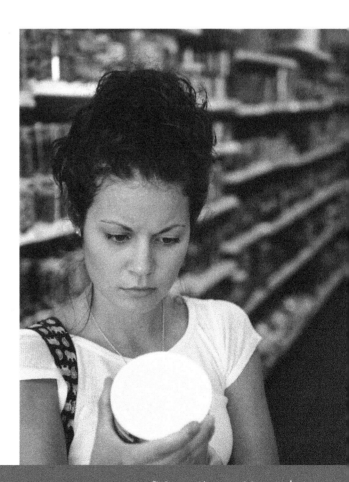

I am afraid of gaining too much weight during my pregnancy

Current weight-gain guidelines create a serious dilemma for you during your pregnancy. You are likely to be told, on the one hand, "Don't gain too much weight," and on the other hand, "Don't diet." Most women gain more or less than the recommended amount, and most women have a healthy baby. But struggling with your eating and weight could undermine your nutrition and health and take away from the joy and wonder of your pregnancy:

- No matter their size to begin with, pregnant women who try to restrict weight gain are more anxious, depressed, angry, stressed, and demoralized.

- Pregnant women who fear obstetrical-visit weight checks don't eat or drink before the visit and try to adjust monthly weight gain based on previous gain.

- Trying to manage weight by eating infrequently increases the risk of preterm delivery as does going without food for prolonged periods.

Being a competent eater supports your pregnancy

Everything about taking good care of yourself with food in every chapter of this booklet applies to you and your pregnancy. Your pattern of weight gain may follow the standard graphs, or it may be unique to you. Your hunger and appetite will vary from month to month, and among the first, second, and third trimesters.

- Feed yourself faithfully. Reliably provide yourself with appealing food at predictable times.

- Connect with your food and your internal cues. Eat as much as you want of food you enjoy.

Trust your body

Pregnancy gives you the priceless opportunity to gain appreciation for your body and for the miracle of giving birth. You can apply everything you have learned in this booklet to:

- Be loving and nurturing with yourself by taking good care of yourself with food.

- Detect and trust information coming from your body to guide your eating.

- Respect and trust your own distinctive pattern of weight gain during pregnancy.

- Develop rewarding and sustainable eating attitudes and behaviors that you can continue after pregnancy and as you raise your child.

Family meals start during pregnancy

If I had a magic wand, I would make eating competence counseling available to all prospective parents. I would help them establish family meals and develop positive eating attitudes and behaviors that are likely to persist after their baby arrives. I have done such counseling with lots of parents-in-waiting and have found them to be delightful in their commitment to their babies. They most often arrive doubting that they are eating well and leave recognizing that they are doing lots better than they thought. We almost always do a bit of tweaking, but it is limited, both because little change is necessary and because it isn't practical or kind to do major surgery on eating.

Eating after the baby

Whether you are breast- or formula-feeding, you have to eat. This goes for fathers as well as mothers. You need your strength, endurance, and emotional steadiness in order to be good parents. When you are hungry, you will be worn out, cranky, and discouraged.

Address challenges to your being a competent eater

You will be so busy at first that it is hard to find time for a meal. Courage! Take care of your body and trust it to carry you through this challenging time.

- Remember to eat. Depend on structure to anchor and remind you to take care of yourself.

- Have easy-to-prepare meals with food you enjoy. Review chapter 5 for ideas. Eat until you feel satisfied. Stop. Do it again the next meal or snack. And the next.

- Trust your body and give it time to adjust to its non-pregnant weight. Don't diet.

Eat (and drink) to support breastfeeding

It is hard to know the extent to which what and how much you eat affects breastmilk quantity and composition. Depend on your being a competent eater to guide you.

- Have regular meals and snacks and eat as much as you want of food you enjoy.

- Remember to drink water. Sit down with a glass of water when you feed your baby.

- Don't skimp on fat. You need it for calories and for making your food taste good.

- Eat a variety of fats. The fat in your breastmilk reflects the fat in your diet and gives your baby the essential fatty acids s/he needs for brain and nervous system development.

- Keep an eye on your weight. If you lose no more than a half pound a week, you are probably eating enough.

Do troubleshooting if your milk supply seems low

Do any of these patterns describe yours? Before you stop breastfeeding, seek help from a professional who will support and preserve your being competent with eating.

- Low weight gain during pregnancy for whatever reason.

- Erratic and unpredictable meals and snacks.

- Having a long list of foods to avoid.

Do troubleshooting if your baby seems upset by something you eat

Traces of anything you eat show up in your breastmilk. Most babies don't mind. A few react. All babies have an immature digestive system. Intestinal gas means the system is working!

- Up to 20% of babies under age 3 months have "unexplained fussiness." Time may be the only cure.

- A small percentage of breastfed infants show allergic symptoms when you eat certain foods: They eat poorly, develop skin rashes, and vomit or have diarrhea.

- Balance your needs and your baby's needs. This is rare, but your baby may be so allergic that it is hard for you to eat enough to be healthy. You may find you need to drink a hypoallergenic formula, or you may have to consider weaning your baby to a hypoallergenic formula.

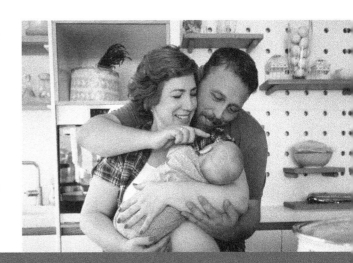

I might have an eating disorder

This booklet is a lifeboat in a sea of distorted eating attitudes and behaviors. Almost everyone feels conflicted and anxious about what and/or how much they eat. Almost everyone repeatedly or continually restricts the amount or type of food they eat to be "healthy" or to keep their weight down. (And talks about it in tedious detail.) As a result of food restriction, many people binge-eat to some extent. The distorted eating attitudes and behaviors that go along with food restriction always take a toll, but they take a *big* toll when eating and not-eating become your life's focus.

Why be concerned?

Having an eating disorder represents a loss in your finding joy in life and being all you can be. An eating disorder can interfere with your physical, emotional, and social health. Your weight may go so low that you have trouble feeling and thinking: You can't organize, study, socialize, and sleep. Your life may be a painful existence that revolves around food and exercise. Rather than being a source of pleasure and self-nurturing, eating or not-eating becomes negative, exaggerated, and handicapping.

Do you put emotional pressure on your eating?

Whether or not you have an eating disorder depends on whether your physical, social, and/or emotional health are impaired. Being overwhelmed and out of control with your eating can look and feel like binge eating disorder. Even if your weight is high or in the "normal" range, keeping it artificially low *for you* can look and feel like anorexia nervosa, as can a sudden or rapid weight loss. Eating attitudes and behaviors centered around other concerns can go to rigid extremes and feel like eating disorders. Consider extreme food selectivity and aversion to unfamiliar food tastes and textures, intense restriction and obsession with eating only "healthy food," anxiety about eating to maintain wellness, dread of choking or vomiting, or extreme fear of eating foods that could cause an allergic reaction.

When to get help with your eating

Whether or not you *call* it an eating disorder, get help if you are upset, rigid, and immobilized with respect to your eating. Find a professional who is proficient with eating competence and has worked with people who struggle with distortions in eating attitudes and behaviors. If you check one or more of these boxes, you really *do* need help—and you are entitled to it.

❑ Your concerns about your weight or about what to eat/not eat affect your relationships with other people.

❑ You see "successfully" managing your eating and weight as central to your life satisfaction.

❑ The chapter 2 connecting-with-eating strategies are too upsetting and overwhelming for you.

❑ The feelings that come up when you tune in to your eating are so scary and upsetting that you just can't tolerate them.

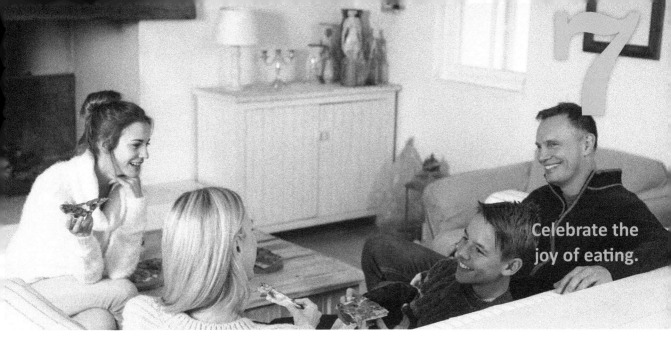
Celebrate the joy of eating.

7

Know what you have learned

This booklet helps you help yourself to become competent with eating. I hope by now you have discovered the joys and rewards of trusting yourself and taking good care of yourself with food.

- You feed yourself faithfully and consistently. You manage your time, eating, and drinking to arrive at meals and snacks hungry and ready to eat.

- You are comfortable with food and with eating.

- You take an interest in food and are relaxed about unfamiliar food.

- You intuitively eat the amount you need and accept the body you get when you do that.

From then to now

- When you started working your way through this booklet, you may have been experiencing some conflict and anxiety about eating. If all has gone well for you, with the help of this booklet you were able to resolve your issues on your own.

- You helped your body learn to eat by connecting with the process of eating.

- You adjusted your attitudes about food by learning to resist interference and get the good-food-bad-food monkey off your back.

- You developed strategies for feeding yourself.

- You discovered you could depend on your being a competent eater to solve eating problems.

What happens next

Holding steady with being a competent eater in our eating- and weight-obsessed culture is difficult. The best you have going for you are the joy of eating and trust in your body to guide you. That joy and trust require nurturing. Life isn't perfect, and at times you may become casual about providing for yourself and connecting with your food. Then your old eating attitudes and behaviors will come back. But when things calm down, you can go back to feeding yourself faithfully and giving yourself permission to eat and your competence with eating will come back. Eventually, you will get to the point where you can use your self-care with eating to help carry you through the tough times.

You may not like what you have learned

It may not have gone so well for you. Rather than feeling joyful and rewarded, taking this deep dive into your eating attitudes and behaviors may have left you feeling more conflicted and anxious than ever. You may discover you have an eating disorder, or you may not. Either way, you can feel better. Work with an eating-competence savvy professional who has experience addressing established and complicated eating problems.

Get help with your eating

I prefer that you have in-person help from a local professional who has been mentored and trained by the Ellyn Satter Institute (ESI). But professionals who understand and properly apply the Satter Eating Competence Model and the Satter division of responsibility in feeding are currently a select group, so ESI offers virtual coaching services. Through questionnaires, videos, and discussion, ESI faculty members and associates can connect with you by computer to help you learn to eat

competently. You can find ESI coaching at *https://www.ellynsatterinstitute.org/*

Find out what holds true for you

To understand your particular challenges with eating, your eating competence coach needs to do an assessment to help you find out what holds true for you. Then you and s/he can put it all together and follow a treatment plan that works. Here is what, together, you and s/he need to consider:

- Your eating attitudes and behaviors.

- Your history with food and eating.

- Your medical history, lifetime weight patterns, and likely disrupters (such as illness, dieting, extreme activity, and weight regain).

- Your current situation and challenges with food and eating.

- Your overall life satisfaction and indications for psychotherapy referral.

Reach out to others

Has this booklet been helpful to you? Would you like others to be helped to feel joyful and relaxed about eating? Here is what you can do:

- Tell a friend about it. Buy them a copy.

- Tell your health professional about it. Encourage them to purchase in bulk for their office.

- Tell your nutrition, health, or wellness teacher about it. Encourage them to purchase in bulk and use it as part of their curriculum.

- Talk about it on social media. Share your experience of becoming competent with eating and addressing your eating problems.

We are at the end of our *Feeding with Love and Good Sense* series. My hope for you is that you have discovered the joy of eating and the joy of feeding your child. Each builds on the other. When you follow the division of responsibility in feeding, your child introduces you to the possibilities of healthy and normal eating. When you go through the motions of feeding yourself faithfully and giving yourself permission to eat, you discover with your very being what healthy and normal eating is all about. It is like being reborn. Embrace the process. Do the work. Trust yourself to learn and grow.

CPSIA information can be obtained
at www.ICGtesting.com
Printed in the USA
LVHW072302080920
R16208700001B/R162087PG664852LVX1B/1

9 780967 118994